OSTEOPHATHIC MANIPULATION THERAPYCRANIOSACRAL THERAPY

Exploring Foundations, Techniques, And Innovations In Holistic Medicine For Every Practitioner

WILFREDO CARSON

INTRODUCTION

Osteopathic Manipulation Therapy (OMT) is a unique type of manual treatment used by osteopathic physicians to diagnose, treat, and prevent a variety of musculoskeletal problems. Unlike traditional medicine, OMT takes a holistic approach to healthcare, taking into account the interconnectivity of the body's structures and functions. This therapy uses expert manipulation of the musculoskeletal system, which includes joints, muscles, and bones, to boost the body's inherent healing potential. OMT is based on the ideas of osteopathy, a medical philosophy developed in the late nineteenth century by Andrew Taylor Still, the founder of osteopathic medicine. This article investigates the historical evolution of OMT, its key ideas, and its critical significance in modern healthcare.

<u>About Therapeutic Manual Therapy.</u>

Osteopathic Manipulation Therapy, often known as osteopathic manipulative treatment (OMT), is a hands-on approach to healthcare that uses physical techniques to improve the body's structure and function. Osteopathic physicians (DOs) use their hands to diagnose and treat a variety of medical disorders, with a focus on the musculoskeletal system and other interrelated systems in the body. The core theory of OMT is based on the belief that the body has an inbuilt potential to heal itself and that by correcting musculoskeletal abnormalities, practitioners may help this natural healing process.

OMT techniques may include soft tissue manipulation, stretching, resistance, and rhythmic joint motions. Practitioners of OMT receive specialized training to develop a great sense of touch and palpation skills that allow them to detect tiny changes in the musculoskeletal system. OMT attempts to restore mobility, relieve pain, and improve overall function through targeted manual interventions. This therapy is utilized not just to treat musculoskeletal diseases, but also to manage a variety of medical difficulties, including respiratory and circulatory disorders.

Historical Development of OMT

Osteopathic Manipulation Therapy dates back to the late nineteenth century when Dr. Andrew Taylor Still, a frontier physician, created osteopathic medicine. Dr. Still's unhappiness with standard medical techniques at the time, along with a thorough understanding of anatomy and physiology, led him to develop a novel approach to healing. He explained the basics of osteopathy, emphasizing the interdependence of the musculoskeletal system and an individual's entire health.

In 1874, Dr. Still established the fundamental concepts of osteopathy, laying the cornerstone for OMT. He argued that structural disruptions in the body, particularly in the musculoskeletal system, could cause a variety of diseases and health problems. Dr. Still was convinced that by manipulating the musculoskeletal system, physicians might restore balance and allow the body to recover itself. This holistic approach differed from the dominant medical methods of the period, which frequently depended on drugs and intrusive procedures.

Dr. Still founded the American School of Osteopathy in Kirksville, Missouri, in 1892, thereby establishing osteopathic medicine. This organization established the first osteopathic medical school, offering instruction and training to those aspiring to become osteopathic physicians.

The curriculum covered osteopathy principles, anatomy, and practical approaches for diagnosing and treating a variety of ailments. Osteopathic medicine became increasingly popular throughout time, and more osteopathic medical schools were created around the United States.

As OMT evolved, several osteopathic organizations were founded to encourage research, education, and the standardization of professional standards. The American Osteopathic Association (AOA), founded in 1897, was instrumental in expanding the science and lobbying for the acceptance of osteopathic medicine. OMT progressively gained acceptability in the larger medical community, and osteopathic practitioners became an essential component of the healthcare system.

The Importance of OMT in Modern Healthcare

Osteopathic Manipulation Therapy is extremely important in modern medicine for a variety of reasons. One of OMT's significant accomplishments is its comprehensive approach to patient care.

Unlike conventional medicine, which generally focuses on symptom management, OMT targets the root causes of health problems by taking into account the interconnection of the body's systems. This approach is consistent with the rising realization of the necessity of treating patients as entire people, rather than discrete symptoms.

OMT is particularly useful in the treatment of musculoskeletal problems, which range from acute accidents to chronic conditions. Osteopathic physicians use hands-on procedures to identify and treat structural imbalances, limitations, or dysfunctions in the musculoskeletal system. This not only alleviates pain and increases mobility, but it also promotes long-term musculoskeletal health.

OMT is frequently used in treatment programs for problems like back pain, neck discomfort, arthritis, and sports injuries.

Another facet of the importance of OMT is its involvement in pain management. Osteopathic physicians are educated to assess and treat pain comprehensively, taking into account both the physical and emotional elements of the patient. By addressing musculoskeletal abnormalities, OMT can help to reduce pain without relying exclusively on drugs. This is consistent with the broader healthcare goals of reducing opioid use and promoting non-pharmacological alternatives to pain management.

OMT has also shown efficacy in improving the respiratory and circulatory systems.

The manual techniques used in OMT can increase rib cage mobility, lung function, and blood flow. This has consequences for asthma, chronic obstructive pulmonary disease (COPD), and heart disease. Osteopathic practitioners may include OMT in their overall therapy of various illnesses to supplement established medical techniques.

Furthermore, OMT is known for its potential to improve patients' general well-being.

The hands-on nature of OMT encourages a therapeutic relationship between the practitioner and the patient.

This individualized approach enables osteopathic practitioners to evaluate not just the physical components of health, but also the patient's lifestyle, stressors, and emotional state. By addressing these aspects, OMT helps to create a more holistic and patient-centered style of therapy.

Osteopathic Manipulation Therapy has grown from Dr. Andrew Taylor Still's visionary discoveries into a well-established and essential component of modern healthcare. Its historical growth, founded on a holistic concept, has prepared the path for a distinct approach to patient treatment.

OMT's importance in modern healthcare stems from its comprehensive character, efficacy in musculoskeletal management, role in pain reduction, and possible effects on respiratory and circulatory health. As osteopathic medicine advances, OMT remains a crucial tool for clinicians to promote health, healing, and overall well-being.

CHAPTER 1
FOUNDATIONS OF OSTEOPATHIC MEDICINE

Osteopathic Medicine is a unique discipline of healthcare that emphasizes a comprehensive approach to patient care, recognizing the interconnection of the body's structure and function. The profession began in the late nineteenth century, when Andrew Taylor Still, the pioneer of osteopathy, proposed a new perspective on the relationship between musculoskeletal integrity and total health. At the heart of Osteopathic Medicine is the belief that the body has the natural power to cure itself given the correct conditions. This fundamental premise governs osteopathic physicians' work, focusing on treating the underlying causes of sickness rather than simply soothing symptoms.

<u>Principles of Osteopathic Medicine</u>

Osteopathic Medicine is founded on four key concepts that guide the thought and practice of osteopathic practitioners. The first concept, "body is a unit," emphasizes the interdependence of the body's many systems. Osteopathic physicians see the body as a dynamic, interconnected whole, with dysfunction in one portion affecting other sections. The second principle, "the body is capable of self-regulation, self-healing, and health maintenance," is consistent with the concept that the body has a natural ability to recover and maintain equilibrium. Osteopathic physicians seek to assist and support the body's intrinsic healing potential.

The third concept, "structure and function are reciprocally interrelated," underlines the musculoskeletal system's close relationship to the body's physiological activities. Osteopathic doctors understand that structural changes, such as misalignments or limitations, can impair normal function and contribute to disease. In contrast, improving the body's structure can improve its ability to function optimally. The fourth principle, "rational treatment is based on an understanding of the basic principles of body unity, self-regulation, and the interrelationship of structure and function," informs osteopathic practitioners' diagnostic and therapeutic techniques. It emphasizes the necessity of viewing the patient as a whole and personalizing treatment to address the root causes of sickness.

Osteopathic Philosophy and Approach to Healthcare.

The philosophy of Osteopathic Medicine goes beyond the four essential principles to provide a broader perspective on health and disease. Osteopathic practitioners utilize a patient-centered approach that considers the individual's specific circumstances, lifestyle, and surroundings. This personalized approach reflects the notion that healthcare should be adapted to each patient's particular needs, recognizing the wide range of factors that influence health.

The concept of "somatic dysfunction" is essential to osteopathic philosophy. It refers to defective or altered function of the musculoskeletal system, which includes the linked nerves, blood vessels, and other systems. Osteopathic practitioners think that somatic dysfunction can lead to a variety of health problems and that treating it is critical for restoring maximum health. The hands-on treatment technique of Osteopathic Manipulative Therapy (OMT) is critical in detecting and addressing somatic dysfunction.

In addition to somatic dysfunction, osteopathic philosophy recognizes the importance of the patient's mental, emotional, and social well-being. Osteopathic physicians understand the complex connection between the mind and body, and how psychological problems can affect physical health and vice versa. This holistic approach is consistent with

pg. 17

the biopsychosocial model of healthcare, which emphasizes the interdependence of biological, psychological, and social elements in diagnosing and treating illness.

Key Concepts of Osteopathic Manipulative Therapy

Osteopathic Manipulative Therapy (OMT) is a unique feature of Osteopathic Medicine that includes a variety of hands-on approaches for evaluating and treating somatic dysfunction. These procedures, which are performed by experienced osteopathic physicians, include expert palpation, manipulation, and mobilization of the musculoskeletal system. The fundamental ideas of OMT focus on the body's ability to heal itself, the interplay between structure and function, and the restoration of balance for optimal health.

OMT is based on the belief that the body has an innate potential to self-regulate and heal. Osteopathic practitioners use a variety of OMT treatments to help the body's natural healing process by correcting musculoskeletal constraints or imbalances. These hands-on therapies aim to restore circulation, nerve function, and overall tissue health, encouraging the body's ability to heal from within.

Another important notion in OMT is the link between structure and function. Osteopathic physicians use their knowledge of anatomy and physiology to identify musculoskeletal dysfunctions. This may include an assessment of joint mobility, muscle tension, and general body alignment. OMT uses focused manipulation and mobilization to restore ideal structure and, as a result, improve physiological function. This approach is consistent with the osteopathic principle that the body's structure and function are inextricably linked.

OMT techniques are varied and adaptive, ranging from direct procedures involving particular joint movements to indirect techniques that focus on reducing tension in surrounding tissues. Direct treatments may include high-velocity, low-amplitude thrusts to restore joint mobility, whereas indirect techniques frequently incorporate gentle stretches and soft tissue manipulation to promote relaxation and realignment. Osteopathic practitioners adjust their approach to each patient's situation, taking into account age, health status, and personal preferences.

The use of OMT goes beyond the treatment of musculoskeletal problems. Osteopathic physicians understand the possible effects of somatic dysfunction on numerous organ systems and general health. Practitioners of OMT seek to address not only localized musculoskeletal issues but also the larger repercussions of somatic dysfunction on the body's physiological and neurological systems. This comprehensive approach reflects Osteopathic Medicine's holistic character and emphasis on addressing the underlying causes of sickness.

The basics of osteopathic medicine are a unique set of beliefs and philosophies that define the profession's approach to treatment. Osteopathic practitioners believe in the body's innate ability to self-regulate and heal. Osteopathic Medicine is founded on the ideas of body unity, self-regulation, structure-function interaction, and rational treatment. The idea extends to a patient-centered approach, which recognizes the significance of individual circumstances, lifestyle, and the mind-body connection in treatment.

Osteopathic Manipulative Therapy (OMT) emerges as a critical component of Osteopathic Medicine, embracing the notions of the body's self-healing capacity and the interdependence of structure and function. OMT treatments, which range from direct joint manipulations to indirect soft tissue mobilizations, are intended to discover and correct somatic dysfunction. This hands-on approach not only tackles musculoskeletal disorders but also acknowledges the larger impact of somatic dysfunction on overall health. OMT emphasizes the holistic character of Osteopathic Medicine by offering a distinct and tailored approach to patient care.

CHAPTER 2
ANATOMY AND PHYSIOLOGY FOR OMT

In the field of Osteopathic Manipulative Therapy (OMT), a thorough grasp of human anatomy and physiology serves as the foundation for efficient therapeutic intervention. The musculoskeletal system, which includes bones, muscles, joints, and connective tissues, is inextricably tied to OMT's ideas and methods. The musculoskeletal system review dives into the structural underpinning that supports the body, emphasizing how bones and muscles work together to ensure stability, movement, and general physiological balance.

Practitioners of OMT must be well-versed in skeletal anatomy to understand the dynamics of joint function and potential sources of dysfunction. Understanding the biomechanics of joints and the linkages between various musculoskeletal components is critical for accurate diagnosis and tailored therapy interventions. Furthermore, a deep understanding of the musculoskeletal system helps osteopathic practitioners detect subtle changes in structure and function that may be underlying patients' complaints, allowing for a more comprehensive approach to therapy.

Neuroanatomy related to OMT:

The complex interaction between the neurological system and Osteopathic

Manipulative Therapy emphasizes the importance of neuroanatomy in this treatment technique.

The nervous system, which includes both central and peripheral components, is essential for coordinating body activities and responding to external stimuli. OMT practitioners study neuroanatomy to better understand the complex brain networks that underlie motor control, sensory perception, and autonomic processes.

Neuroanatomy is especially essential to OMT because it reinforces the concept of somatic dysfunction, which is a fundamental component of osteopathic philosophy. Somatic dysfunction is defined as the impaired or changed function of associated somatic (body framework) system components such as the skeletal, arthrodial, and myofascial tissues. With a thorough understanding of neuroanatomy, OMT practitioners can decipher the neurophysiological basis of somatic dysfunction, allowing them to develop therapies that target not only the musculoskeletal aspects but also the neurological components that contribute to dysfunction.

Furthermore, the neuroanatomical approach in OMT incorporates the concept of neuroplasticity, which emphasizes the nervous system's adaptability. Osteopathic practitioners use this knowledge to promote nutriregulation, attempting to restore optimal function and relieve symptoms using physical treatments. The incorporation of neuroanatomy into OMT therapy ensures a thorough understanding of the complex link between the musculoskeletal and neurological systems, promoting a holistic approach to patient care.

The significance of understanding body mechanics:

The substantial impact of body mechanics on health and well-being highlights the need to incorporate this notion into the practice of Osteopathic Manipulative Therapy (OMT). Body mechanics is the coordinated action of muscles, joints, and other musculoskeletal systems during movement and posture.

A thorough understanding of body mechanics is essential for OMT practitioners because it serves as the foundation for diagnosing biomechanical dysfunctions and developing focused therapeutic interventions.

OMT lays a strong emphasis on restoring optimal body mechanics to relieve pain, improve mobility, and enhance general function. Practitioners who understand the complexities of body mechanics can evaluate how deviations from normal movement patterns contribute to musculoskeletal dysfunction. OMT attempts to restore balance and functionality by identifying areas with compromised biomechanics and using manual approaches that target specific structures and tissues.

Furthermore, the use of body mechanics in OMT goes beyond the treatment room by stressing patient education on ergonomics, posture, and movement patterns. Osteopathic practitioners provide their patients with the knowledge and techniques they need to maintain good body mechanics in their daily activities, preventing musculoskeletal disorders from recurring and encouraging long-term health.

Understanding body mechanics connects with biomechanical principles such as equilibrium and stability. OMT therapies frequently focus on restoring balance in the musculoskeletal system and correcting asymmetries and dysfunctions that can jeopardize stability. OMT practitioners use precise manual techniques to improve proprioception and neuromuscular coordination, which leads to better body mechanics and total functional capacity.

The confluence of anatomy, neuroanatomy, and body mechanics is the foundation of Osteopathic Manipulative Therapy.

A thorough understanding of the musculoskeletal system serves as the anatomical foundation for OMT treatment, allowing practitioners to identify structural nuances and treat dysfunctions. Neuroanatomy improves OMT by illuminating the neurological basis of somatic dysfunction and emphasizing the nervous system's plasticity. Simultaneously, a thorough grasp of body mechanics enables OMT practitioners to identify and intervene in biomechanical dysfunctions, supporting optimal function and equipping patients with the knowledge needed to maintain musculoskeletal health. Together, these ideas contribute to the holistic and patient-centered approach that distinguishes Osteopathic Manipulative Therapy.

CHAPTER 3
TECHNIQUES IN OSTEOPATHIC MANIPULATION

Osteopathic Manipulation Therapy (OMT) refers to a group of treatments used to diagnose and treat musculoskeletal disorders by modifying the body's structure. This therapy technique is based on osteopathic concepts, which highlight the body's interconnection and natural ability to repair itself. The approaches used in OMT are roughly classified as direct and indirect methods, with each serving a specific role in resolving dysfunction and increasing overall health.

Direct approaches in OMT entail delivering force to specific body locations to restore normal function.

Soft tissue techniques involve manipulating muscles, tendons, and ligaments to relieve stress, increase flexibility, and promote circulation. Practitioners may use treatments such as myofascial release, trigger point therapy, and deep tissue massage.

These procedures attempt to break down adhesions, minimize muscular spasms, and improve soft tissue mobility.

High-velocity, Low-Amplitude (HVLA) Thrust Techniques are a dynamic feature of OMT. This procedure comprises fast, controlled movements applied to joints, which frequently result in an audible "pop" or "crack." The sound is caused by the expulsion of gas bubbles within the joint, which creates a temporary vacuum. HVLA procedures are frequently utilized to relieve joint limitations, increase the range of motion, and restore optimal joint function. Although the mechanism behind the "pop" is not entirely understood, the therapeutic advantages are thought to be due to joint mobilization and proprioceptive stimulation.

Muscle Energy Techniques (MET) involve the patient actively resisting or contracting certain muscles as the practitioner administers counterforce. This collaborative endeavor aims to enhance muscle function, joint mobility, and musculoskeletal balance. MET can be used to treat a variety of conditions, including muscular imbalances, joint constraints, and postural irregularities. The participatory nature of MET allows for a customized approach, tailoring the treatment to each patient's specific requirements and talents.

Indirect strategies in OMT aim to improve the body's ability to self-correct and heal by working with, rather than against, its natural processes. Myofascial Release is an important indirect technique that focuses on the fascial system, which surrounds and pervades muscles, bones, and organs. Practitioners apply gentle, persistent pressure to the fascia to remove limitations, restore flexibility, improve tissue mobility, and relieve pain. Myofascial release is particularly useful for treating chronic illnesses and promoting structural equilibrium.

Counterstain is another indirect technique that involves finding painful areas linked to musculoskeletal dysfunction and relieving strain through a passive, pain-free stance.

The goal is to reset the neuromuscular system, reducing tension and facilitating normal function. Counterstain is regarded as a gentle and non-invasive approach, making it appropriate for a wide spectrum of patients, even those experiencing acute pain or sensitivity.

LAST addresses dysfunction in ligaments and joint capsules. Practitioners utilize gentle, controlled movements to relieve tension in these structures, increase joint mobility, and restore appropriate function.

LAST is commonly used in circumstances where ligamentous and joint capsule involvement causes pain and restricted movement. LAST attempts to improve total musculoskeletal health by increasing balance and flexibility in these connective tissues.

Osteopathic Manipulation Therapy includes a variety of techniques, both direct and indirect, each with a distinct aim in treating musculoskeletal problems. Soft Tissue procedures, HVLA Thrust Techniques, and Muscle Energy Techniques are examples of direct procedures that include physically manipulating tissues and joints to restore normal function. Indirect treatments, such as Myofascial Release, Counterstrain, and Ligamentous Articular Strain Technique, use the body's healing processes to promote self-correction and overall health. Integrating these approaches enables osteopathic practitioners to deliver comprehensive and patient-centered care, addressing a wide range of musculoskeletal disorders while also contributing to their patients' overall health.

CHAPTER 4
OMT FOR SPECIFIC CONDITIONS

Osteopathic Manipulative Therapy (OMT) has been used for a variety of ailments, demonstrating its adaptability and efficacy across multiple medical areas. OMT is an important tool for treating musculoskeletal diseases such as joint pain, muscular strain, and structural misalignment. Osteopathic practitioners use a hands-on approach to restore musculoskeletal balance and function, including soft tissue manipulation, stretching, and joint mobilization. This tailored technique not only relieves pain but also strengthens the body's inherent healing capabilities.

In the context of neurological illnesses, OMT provides a novel therapeutic method for treating nervous system issues.

Osteopathic physicians use procedures to increase the flow of cerebrospinal fluid and neuronal function. This includes cranial osteopathy, a subset of OMT that focuses on the delicate movements of the skull and cranial sutures. Practitioners use gentle manipulations to improve the function of the central nervous system, potentially affecting diseases such as migraines, tension headaches, and some neurological dysfunctions.

OMT therapies are beneficial to both respiratory and cardiovascular problems. Osteopathic physicians understand the interdependence of the body's systems and use procedures to improve respiratory and cardiovascular health.

OMT can improve rib movement, lung expansion, and diaphragmatic function, all of which contribute to increased respiratory efficiency. Additionally, manipulation techniques may be used to improve blood flow, reduce vascular stress, and boost overall cardiovascular health. OMT's integrative character makes it an effective supplement to traditional medical treatments for illnesses such as asthma, chronic obstructive pulmonary disease (COPD), and some cardiovascular disorders.

In the field of obstetrics and Gynecology, OMT is becoming more well-acknowledged for its ability to improve women's health throughout their reproductive lifetimes.

Osteopathic physicians use mild treatments to correct structural abnormalities and improve pelvic alignment. This is especially useful during pregnancy, when OMT may help ease typical discomforts such as back pain, pelvic pain, and sciatica. OMT may also help to facilitate proper fetal positioning and ease the childbirth process. Postpartum, OMT can help with the healing of musculoskeletal alterations and improve the mother's overall well-being.

The incorporation of OMT into the care of specific illnesses exemplifies the osteopathic idea of treating the full person rather than merely symptoms. By treating structural and functional abnormalities, OMT seeks to improve the body's natural ability to recover and maintain health. As OMT evolves, new research and clinical trials add to the expanding body of evidence supporting its efficacy in a variety of medical fields.

OMT for Musculoskeletal Disorders

Osteopathic Manipulative Therapy (OMT) is an important therapeutic technique in the management of musculoskeletal disorders, which include a wide range of illnesses affecting the bones, joints, muscles, and connective tissues. Osteopathic physicians use a holistic approach, taking into account the musculoskeletal system's interconnectivity to other body systems. OMT in musculoskeletal problems aims to restore structural integrity, increase mobility, and relieve pain with hands-on manipulations.

One of the fundamental foundations of OMT for musculoskeletal illnesses is the concept of somatic dysfunction, which refers to the impaired or altered function of linked musculoskeletal components. Osteopathic physicians conduct detailed exams to identify areas of somatic dysfunction and use several treatments to treat these problems. Soft tissue manipulation, joint articulation, and myofascial release are among the various manipulative techniques used to treat specific musculoskeletal issues.

Soft tissue manipulation is the process of applying pressure and stretching to muscles, tendons, and ligaments to relieve tension and increase flexibility. This treatment is particularly useful for muscle spasms, strains, and myofascial pain syndromes. By targeting soft tissue constraints, OMT attempts to improve blood flow, reduce inflammation, and promote natural healing.

Another important aspect of OMT for musculoskeletal problems is joint articulation, which focuses on enhancing joint range of motion and function. Osteopathic physicians mobilize joints with precise movements that alleviate limitations and promote healthy biomechanics. This method is useful in situations such as osteoarthritis, where joint movement may be limited.

Myofascial release is a technique for treating the fascial system, which is a network of connective tissues that surrounds and supports muscles, bones, and organs. Osteopathic physicians utilize gentle sustained pressure to relieve fascial limitations, which promotes tissue mobility and reduces pain. Myofascial release is very important in disorders like fibromyalgia and chronic pain syndromes.

The use of OMT in musculoskeletal problems extends to sports medicine, where athletes frequently seek osteopathic care for injury prevention and recovery. Osteopathic practitioners may employ OMT to correct biomechanical imbalances, increase joint mobility, and optimize muscle function, all of which contribute to better sports performance and lower injury risk.

OMT in musculoskeletal problems illustrates the osteopathic dedication to a comprehensive, patient-centered approach. OMT seeks to restore balance and function to the musculoskeletal system by addressing somatic dysfunction using a variety of manipulative techniques, offering effective treatment for a wide range of disorders. Ongoing research and clinical trials continue to advance our understanding and refining of OMT in the context of musculoskeletal health.

OMT for Neurological Disorders

Osteopathic Manipulative Therapy (OMT) was developed as a separate treatment method in the field of neurological disorders, providing a unique collection of interventions aimed at optimizing neural function and treating nervous system problems. Osteopathic physicians understand the complex link between the musculoskeletal and neurological systems, and they use hands-on manipulations to impact the function of the central nervous system (CNS) and relieve symptoms associated with a variety of neurological disorders.

Cranial osteopathy is a unique type of OMT that focuses on the skull and its delicate movements.

Osteopathic clinicians think that the cranial bones move rhythmically and that abnormalities in this motion may contribute to neurological dysfunction. Practitioners use mild and precise manipulations to restore normal cranial mobility and impact CNS function. Cranial osteopathy is frequently used in the treatment of migraines, tension headaches, and certain neurological problems.

In addition to cranial osteopathy, OMT employs procedures to improve the flow of cerebrospinal fluid (CSF) throughout the central nervous system. The correct circulation of CSF is critical for the health and function of the CNS. Osteopathic physicians use treatments like myofascial release and soft tissue manipulation to treat limitations that may be preventing CSF flow. OMT improves the mobility of the tissues around the spine and skull, which adds to overall nervous system health.

OMT therapies may help neuropathies, radiculopathies, and certain functional neurological diseases. Osteopathic practitioners customize their approach to each patient's specific needs, taking into account the differences between neurological conditions. OMT is a beneficial addition to standard neurological care since it addresses somatic dysfunction while also optimizing neural function.

The holistic character of OMT is consistent with the osteopathic idea of treating the entire person. In the case of neurological illnesses, this approach includes not just symptom treatment but also an examination of the underlying structural and functional abnormalities that may contribute to neurological symptoms. Ongoing research in the field investigates the processes by which OMT affects the nervous system, adding to the expanding body of evidence supporting its efficacy in neurological care.

OMT in neurological illnesses exemplifies the osteopathic dedication to a complete, patient-centered approach. OMT provides a unique therapy option for people suffering from a variety of neurological diseases by merging specialized approaches such as cranial osteopathy and addressing cerebrospinal fluid dynamics. As our understanding of the complicated interactions within the nervous system grows, OMT is set to play an increasingly important role in the integrated treatment of neurological illnesses.

<u>OMT for Respiratory and Cardiovascular Conditions.</u>

Osteopathic Manipulative Therapy (OMT) appears as a significant adjuvant in the therapy of respiratory and cardiovascular problems, demonstrating its versatility in treating both musculoskeletal and systemic issues. Osteopathic physicians understand the interdependence of the body's systems and use manipulative techniques to improve respiratory and cardiovascular health. OMT improves pulmonary and circulatory efficiency by utilizing soft tissue manipulation, rib mobilization, and diaphragmatic methods.

OMT can help improve lung function and address musculoskeletal causes of respiratory discomfort. Soft tissue manipulation is used to relieve tension in the respiratory muscles, allowing for more chest wall mobility and diaphragmatic expansion. Osteopathic physicians may also use rib mobilization procedures to increase rib cage expansion and improve lung ventilation. Asthma, chronic obstructive pulmonary disease (COPD), and respiratory infections may benefit from OMT's integrative approach in addition to standard medical interventions.

Rib mobilization is a type of OMT that involves manipulating rib joints and articulations.

This procedure is intended to increase rib mobility and restore normal breathing mechanics. Osteopathic physicians use precise and controlled movements to address rib cage constraints, which may alleviate respiratory symptoms and improve overall lung function. Rib mobility influences respiratory disorders, contributing to OMT's comprehensive approach to addressing systemic health.

In terms of cardiovascular health, OMT may affect vascular function and contribute to the circulatory system's overall health. Manipulative techniques used on the thoracic spine and rib cage might alter the sympathetic and parasympathetic tone, potentially affecting blood pressure regulation. Osteopathic practitioners may use diaphragmatic techniques to improve venous return and lymphatic drainage, hence promoting cardiovascular health.

The particular processes by which OMT affects cardiovascular parameters are still being investigated.

The use of OMT in the care of respiratory and cardiovascular diseases is consistent with the osteopathic philosophy of treating the whole person. OMT attempts to improve total physiological function by targeting both musculoskeletal and systemic variables. As we get a better understanding of the interconnection of physiological systems, OMT will become an increasingly effective therapeutic tool for boosting respiratory and cardiovascular health.

OMT for respiratory and cardiovascular disorders exemplifies the holistic and integrative nature of osteopathic treatment. OMT complements traditional medical interventions by using manipulative techniques that address musculoskeletal and systemic contributors to respiratory and cardiovascular disorders. Ongoing research efforts continue to shed information on the specific processes by which OMT affects respiratory and cardiovascular health, reinforcing its significance in complete patient treatment.

<u>OMT in Obstetrics and Gynecology.</u>

Osteopathic Manipulative Therapy (OMT) is a unique and evolving area in obstetrics and gynecology, providing a comprehensive approach to women's health throughout the reproductive lifecycle. Osteopathic physicians use manipulative treatments to correct structural imbalances, improve pelvic alignment, and alleviate typical musculoskeletal problems related to pregnancy and gynaecological diseases.

During pregnancy, women frequently feel musculoskeletal discomfort such as back pain, pelvic pain, and sciatica. OMT becomes an effective treatment option for these symptoms by addressing changes in posture, weight distribution, and hormonal influences on the musculoskeletal system. Osteopathic physicians utilize mild and precise treatments to improve pelvic biomechanics, reduce muscular tension, and increase overall pregnancy comfort.

OMT in obstetrics focuses on optimizing fetal positioning. Osteopathic physicians understand the importance of fetal presentation during the birthing process and may use procedures to modify the baby's position in the uterus.

By correcting musculoskeletal and ligamentous abnormalities, OMT hopes to establish an environment conducive to good fetal placement, potentially lowering the risk of problems during labor and delivery.

Postpartum, OMT can help with the rehabilitation of musculoskeletal alterations caused by pregnancy and childbirth. Osteopathic physicians treat conditions such as pelvic floor dysfunction, diastasis recti, and structural realignment. By encouraging optimal healing and recovery, OMT assists women in restoring musculoskeletal health after childbirth.

In gynecology, OMT can be used to treat diseases like pelvic discomfort, endometriosis, and menstrual abnormalities.

Osteopathic physicians recognize the interdependence of the musculoskeletal and visceral systems, and that abnormalities in one can lead to symptoms in the other. Practitioners use manipulative techniques to restore balance and function to the pelvic region, which may provide relief for gynaecological disorders.

The use of OMT in obstetrics and gynecology is consistent with the osteopathic idea of treating the entire person. By taking into account the musculoskeletal, visceral, and hormonal elements of women's health, OMT provides an integrative approach to treating a variety of disorders throughout the reproductive lifecycle. OMT's compassionate and patient-centered nature makes it ideal for the specific needs and concerns of women at various phases of life.

OMT in obstetrics and gynecology is a dynamic and expanding aspect of osteopathic medicine. From managing musculoskeletal discomfort during pregnancy to improving fetal placement and promoting postpartum recovery, OMT provides a comprehensive approach to women's health. As research in this field advances, OMT will play an increasingly important role in enhancing women's well-being throughout their reproductive journey.

CHAPTER 6
OMT RESEARCH AND EVIDENCE-BASED PRACTICE

Integrating Osteopathic Manipulative Therapy (OMT) into Clinical Practice necessitates a thorough understanding of patient assessment and diagnosis, strategic treatment planning, and goal setting, as well as the successful integration of OMT into multidisciplinary healthcare systems. This holistic approach to patient care is consistent with the osteopathic philosophy, which emphasizes the interconnection of the body's structure and function. In this context, patient assessment and diagnosis are the foundations of OMT integration, laying the groundwork for individualized treatment programs that address the patient's specific requirements and objectives. As a result, therapy planning and goal setting are critical in improving the therapeutic effects of OMT. Finally, incorporating OMT into multidisciplinary healthcare settings improves its effectiveness by encouraging collaboration among healthcare experts from different disciplines. This conversation delves into each of these principles in depth.

Patient assessment and diagnosis in the context of Osteopathic Manipulative Therapy (OMT) is an important phase that lays the groundwork for a targeted and tailored treatment plan. OMT practitioners use a rigorous and systematic examination approach to analyze the patient's musculoskeletal system, as well as other aspects affecting their overall health. The evaluation frequently begins with a thorough medical history, followed by a physical examination that may include assessing the patient's posture, range of motion, and texture. Palpation, an important aspect of OMT, enables practitioners to detect areas of restricted motion or aberrant tissue tension. This complete assessment helps to diagnose somatic dysfunctions and suggest areas where OMT can be most effective.

The osteopathic approach to patient assessment goes beyond the musculoskeletal system, taking into account the interconnection of other body systems. Practitioners assess a patient's total health, including lifestyle, stresses, and nutritional state.

This comprehensive assessment is consistent with the principles of osteopathic medicine, emphasizing the significance of treating the complete person rather than individual symptoms.

The addition of conventional medical diagnostics, such as imaging investigations and laboratory testing, improves the diagnostic process and ensures a thorough picture of the patient's health status.

Treatment Planning and Goal Setting in OMT entails turning patient evaluation and diagnosis findings into a systematic and tailored treatment plan. OMT practitioners use their knowledge to choose the most appropriate manipulative techniques and methods depending on the detected somatic dysfunctions. The treatment plan specifies the frequency and duration of OMT sessions, taking into account the patient's response to prior treatments and the predicted rate of healing. Furthermore, OMT practitioners work with patients to set realistic and attainable treatment goals.

Goal planning in OMT goes beyond the resolution of specific bodily dysfunctions to include the improvement of general well-being and functional capabilities. Practitioners collaborate with patients to set functional goals such as increased mobility, pain relief, and optimal musculoskeletal function.

The collaborative aspect of goal setting allows patients to actively participate in their healthcare, instilling a sense of ownership and motivation throughout the treatment process. Regular review and goal revision guarantee that the treatment plan evolves in sync with the patient's development and evolving health needs.

Incorporating OMT into Multidisciplinary Healthcare acknowledges the importance of collaborating among healthcare professionals from many disciplines to improve patient care. OMT practitioners collaborate with physicians, physical therapists, and other healthcare professionals to provide a holistic and integrative approach to patient management. Effective communication and shared decision-making are critical in multidisciplinary settings, ensuring that OMT is seamlessly integrated with other elements of patient care.

OMT practitioners collaborate with other healthcare experts by exchanging information about the patient's diagnosis, treatment plan, and progress. This sharing of information allows for a more comprehensive picture of the patient's health, permitting coordinated and complementary interventions. When OMT is included in pain management strategies, collaboration with pain specialists, psychologists, and rehabilitation experts is especially important. This multidisciplinary approach tackles the multidimensional nature of pain while improving the overall efficacy of patient care. The incorporation of OMT into multidisciplinary healthcare contexts includes teaching and training. OMT practitioners regularly contribute to their colleagues' education, promoting a shared understanding of the principles and advantages of osteopathic medicine. Workshops, conferences, and collaborative case discussions give chances for healthcare practitioners to expand their knowledge and skills in OMT. This educational exchange fosters an interdisciplinary culture of respect and cooperation, which benefits patients by providing a more thorough and integrated approach to healthcare.

Integrating Osteopathic Manipulative Therapy into Clinical Practice necessitates a thorough understanding of patient assessment and diagnosis, careful treatment planning and goal setting, and effective teamwork in multidisciplinary healthcare settings.

These ideas all contribute to the comprehensive, patient-centered approach that distinguishes osteopathic medicine. As OMT gains recognition for its usefulness in a variety of clinical situations, its smooth integration into diverse healthcare settings has the potential to improve overall patient outcomes while also contributing to the growth of comprehensive and integrative healthcare practices.

CHAPTER 7
OMT IN SPECIAL POPULATIONS

Osteopathic Manipulative Therapy (OMT) has a long history, founded on osteopathy ideas that emphasize the interdependence of the body's structure and function. The discipline has grown over time, and with advancements in research methodology, there has been a greater emphasis on studying the efficacy and mechanisms of OMT. The overview of OMT research focuses on the wide range of manipulative methods used by osteopathic practitioners and their effects on various health issues.

One aspect of OMT research focuses on understanding the biomechanical and physiological changes caused by manipulative therapies. Researchers used modern imaging tools, such as magnetic resonance imaging (MRI) and ultrasound, to visualize the changes in musculoskeletal structures after OMT. This research seeks to explore the mechanisms by which manual techniques affect tissues, joints, and brain pathways, leading to a more complete understanding of OMT's underlying physiological impacts.

OMT research also includes clinical trials that evaluate the therapeutic efficacy of manipulative therapies in a variety of medical diseases. Randomized controlled trials (RCTs) are critical in assessing the efficacy of OMT vs standard therapies or placebo interventions. These studies not only provide light on the specific situations in which OMT may be beneficial, but they also help to build evidence-based guidelines for its implementation into clinical practice.

OMT's multifaceted character needs a comprehensive study approach that takes into account not only the biomechanical aspects but also the neurophysiological, neuroendocrine, and immunological responses to manual interventions. Integrating these varied perspectives leads to a more comprehensive understanding of how OMT affects the body's homeostasis and self-healing mechanisms. This holistic approach is consistent with the fundamental ideas of osteopathic philosophy, emphasizing the body's intrinsic potential to heal and the significance of treating both symptoms and underlying causes of illness.

As OMT research advances, there is an increasing realization of the importance of standardized outcome measurements and study methodologies. Establishing standard techniques makes it easier to compare findings across studies and increases the dependability of the evidence. This uniformity is critical for establishing a solid foundation of information that may influence therapeutic decisions and contribute to the larger area of manual medicine.

Current Evidence Supporting OMT

The body of evidence supporting OMT has grown dramatically in recent years, now covering a wide range of medical diseases and patient populations. Osteopathic physicians use a variety of manipulative techniques, including soft tissue mobilization, myofascial release, and joint articulation, to address particular dysfunctions discovered during the patient assessment. The present evidence for OMT encompasses a wide range of medical specializations, demonstrating its usefulness across multiple healthcare areas.

OMT is effective in treating musculoskeletal problems by relieving pain, increasing joint mobility, and improving functional outcomes. Numerous clinical research on conditions such as low back pain, osteoarthritis, and neck pain have repeatedly shown that OMT is more effective than traditional treatments. The mechanisms underlying these effects include biomechanical modifications, pain pathway regulation, and the release of endogenous anti-inflammatory mediators.

Beyond musculoskeletal issues, OMT has shown promise in helping to control respiratory illnesses. Studies on the effects of OMT on illnesses such as asthma and chronic obstructive pulmonary disease (COPD) indicate that manipulative therapies may improve respiratory function, reduce dyspnea, and improve overall quality of life. These findings highlight OMT's potential systemic effects, including its ability to alter not only the musculoskeletal but also the respiratory and circulatory systems.

Neurological problems such as tension headaches and migraines have also been studied in the setting of OMT. The available research suggests that manual treatments targeting cranial and cervical regions may help to reduce headache frequency and intensity. The neurophysiological processes underpinning these effects include pain pathway regulation and the release of neurochemicals associated with headache pathogenesis.

In Pediatrics, OMT has attracted interest for its possible involvement in the treatment of disorders such as otitis media and colic. Studies on the application of manipulative methods in paediatric populations suggest that OMT may help to reduce the frequency of ear infections and improve symptoms of gastrointestinal distress. However, further study is needed to determine particular methods and criteria for OMT in paediatric therapy.

While the existing evidence for OMT is strong, ongoing research is helping to improve our understanding of its optimal application and mechanisms of action. The incorporation of OMT into mainstream healthcare necessitates a thorough evidence basis that goes beyond individual illnesses and encompasses the entire spectrum of patient treatment. As the evidence for OMT grows, it becomes increasingly important to spread this knowledge among healthcare practitioners, enabling collaborative efforts to improve patient outcomes.

Future Directions for OMT Research

As OMT establishes itself as an essential component of holistic healthcare, the direction of future research is critical in developing its clinical uses and expanding its evidence basis.

One significant path for future OMT research is to investigate its role in preventive medicine and health promotion. Investigating the effects of manipulative therapies on immunological function, stress resilience, and overall well-being can help to move the paradigm toward proactive, patient-centered care.

The merging of technology and biomechanics is yet another area in OMT research. Wearable sensors, biofeedback devices, and virtual reality advancements provide new opportunities to objectively measure the effects of manipulative interventions and adjust therapies to individual patient reactions. Integrating these technologies into research protocols improves precision in OMT delivery and enables a more tailored approach to patient care.

Furthermore, future OMT research should focus on understanding the long-term impacts of manipulative therapies. While several studies have established short-term effects, establishing the long-term viability of OMT benefits is critical for improving treatment planning and maximizing healthcare expenditures. Longitudinal studies that analyze the long-term effects of OMT on varied patient populations can provide important insights into its role in chronic illness management and preventative care.

Interdisciplinary collaboration is a viable option for OMT research, as it fosters partnerships with other healthcare fields to investigate synergies and complementary treatments. Integrating OMT with disciplines like physical therapy, chiropractic care, and integrative medicine can result in more comprehensive treatment plans and better patient outcomes. Collaborative research endeavors can also close knowledge gaps and provide a more sophisticated understanding of the broader area of manual medicine.

The patient experience and satisfaction with OMT are topics that deserve more focus in future studies. Qualitative studies that investigate patients' opinions, expectations, and preferences regarding OMT can provide important insights into the psychosocial elements of care. Understanding patient-reported outcomes and factors influencing treatment adherence improves patient-centeredness in OMT and informs therapeutic relationship optimization measures.

Finally, future OMT research should focus on the education and training of osteopathic physicians. It is critical to investigate the influence of various training modalities, continuing education programs, and skill development initiatives on OMT practitioners' proficiency and efficacy to sustain high levels of care. Research in this area can help osteopathic physicians improve their curricula, establish accrediting criteria, and pursue continual professional development.

The future of OMT research has tremendous potential to shape the landscape of holistic healthcare. Embracing preventative medicine, utilizing technology, investigating long-term outcomes, developing interdisciplinary collaboration, prioritizing patient experience, and addressing educational aspects are all critical steps that can catapult OMT to a central role in the continuum of care. As OMT advances, continuous research efforts will add not just to the evidence basis supporting its efficacy, but also to the refinement of clinical practices and the incorporation of manual medicine into mainstream healthcare.

CHAPTER 8
ETHICS AND PROFESSIONALISM IN OSTEOPATHIC MEDICINE

Osteopathic Manipulative Therapy (OMT) is a comprehensive approach to healthcare that focuses on the musculoskeletal system and its role in general well-being. Beyond its generic use, OMT is tailored to specific demographics, addressing their individual needs and concerns. This talk will go into OMT in unique groups, focusing on its use in Pediatrics, geriatrics, and athletes suffering from sports injuries.

In pediatrics, OMT is an effective treatment approach that considers children's dynamic growth and development. Pediatric OMT uses gentle and accurate approaches to address musculoskeletal disorders while taking into account the specific anatomy and physiology of growing bodies. Osteopathic paediatric physicians are educated to diagnose and treat a wide range of disorders, including musculoskeletal imbalances, birth trauma, and developmental issues. Torticollis, plagiocephaly, and feeding challenges are some of the issues that OMT for infants can solve. Osteopathic physicians use gentle treatments to support the natural healing processes in a child's body, enabling healthy growth and development.

Moving on to geriatric OMT, the aging population frequently experiences issues with mobility, joint function, and overall musculoskeletal health. Osteopathic geriatric physicians take a patient-centered approach, taking into account the individual's medical history, comorbidities, and functional state. Geriatric OMT seeks to promote joint mobility, reduce discomfort, and improve overall function in the elderly. Gentle stretching, soft tissue manipulation, and joint mobilization are all possible techniques. Osteopathic physicians can also treat age-related illnesses including osteoarthritis and osteoporosis using specific OMT therapies. This strategy aims to improve older individuals' quality of life by enhancing their musculoskeletal health and fostering independence.

In the context of athletes and sports injuries, OMT is critical for both prevention and recovery. Athletes frequently subject their bodies to strenuous physical demands, which increases the likelihood of musculoskeletal ailments. Osteopathic sports medicine specialists are educated to evaluate biomechanics, identify imbalances, and manage musculoskeletal disorders that may contribute to injury. OMT for athletes comprises a variety of techniques such as myofascial release, joint mobilization, and muscle energy procedures. These interventions attempt to improve flexibility, joint function, and biomechanics to reduce the risk of injuries. OMT is also used in the rehabilitation of sports injuries, which promotes speedier recovery and return to peak performance.

OMT in unusual populations highlights the flexibility and adaptability of this holistic

pg. 81

approach to healing. In pediatrics, OMT is designed to meet the special demands of growing bodies, supporting optimal development and treating specific illnesses that afflict infants and children. Geriatric OMT addresses the issues that the aging population faces, to improve musculoskeletal health, pain relief, and general function in older persons. OMT is an important tool for athletes and sports injuries, as it addresses biomechanical abnormalities and optimizes musculoskeletal function. As OMT evolves, its use in certain groups adds to a more holistic and patient-centered approach to healthcare.

CHAPTER 9
CHALLENGES AND CONTROVERSIES IN OMT

Osteopathic Manipulative Therapy (OMT) has garnered both praise and criticism in the healthcare industry. One contentious feature of OMT is the perceived lack of scientific proof backing its usefulness. Skepticism about OMT's basic ideas, such as the concept of somatic dysfunction and the mechanism of action, has sparked controversy among healthcare professionals. Critics contend that the empirical evidence supporting OMT's efficacy is weak when compared to other well-established medical therapies. The lack of established standards and variable terminology in OMT add to the debate, making it difficult to conduct meaningful research and build a globally accepted foundation for the therapy.

Addressing Skepticism and Misconceptions:

In response to criticism and misconceptions about OMT, it is critical to examine the fundamental ideas that support this therapeutic method. OMT is founded on the osteopathic philosophy, which emphasizes the relationship between the musculoskeletal system and general health.

According to practitioners, treating somatic dysfunction, which is defined as impaired or changed function of linked components, improves the body's self-regulatory processes, resulting in better health results. Skepticism stems from a lack of understanding and acceptance of these principles, as well as variety in how OMT is administered by different practitioners.

Education and communication are critical components in resolving these difficulties, with efforts aimed at raising knowledge among healthcare professionals, patients, and the general public about the evidence-based aspects of OMT and its potential advantages.

Legal and Regulatory Concerns in OMT:

The legal and regulatory context surrounding OMT poses additional issues for the sector to address. One notable issue is the variation in licensure criteria for osteopathic physicians and non-physician osteopaths, which results in a lack of standardized control. In some areas, non-physician osteopaths may not be subject to the same strict restrictions as their physician counterparts, creating concerns about patient safety and service quality. Furthermore, acceptance of OMT as a separate therapeutic modality differs among healthcare systems, influencing insurance coverage and compensation for both practitioners and patients. Legal issues arise when seeking to incorporate OMT into traditional medical procedures, as divergent legal frameworks may impede collaboration and interdisciplinary approaches to patient treatment. Navigating these legal and regulatory complexities is critical to guarantee the validity and integration of OMT into the larger healthcare ecosystem.

OMT has numerous obstacles and conflicts that range from the scientific to the legal and regulatory spheres. Addressing these difficulties will need a collaborative effort by the osteopathic community, healthcare professionals, and legislators to lay a firm foundation of evidence-based practice, debunk myths, and harmonize regulatory frameworks. As the profession evolves, fostering collaboration and dialogue will be critical in securing OMT's due role in comprehensive healthcare models.

CHAPTER 10
THE FUTURE OF OSTEOPATHIC MANIPULATIVE THERAPY

Osteopathic Manipulation Therapy (OMT) has a rich history and has changed over time, becoming an essential component of healthcare. As we look into the future of OMT, one of the most important topics to consider is developments in OMT methodologies.

In recent years, there has been a boom of research and innovation targeted at improving and broadening the scope of OMT. New procedures are being created, and old ones are being refined to improve their efficacy.

These developments are motivated not only by technical progress but also by a better knowledge of human anatomy and the interdependence of bodily systems. As the discipline of OMT continues to integrate modern medical knowledge, it has the potential to make substantial contributions to patient care and healthcare outcomes.

Advances in OMT Techniques

Advances in OMT approaches are multidimensional, combining ancient wisdom with modern scientific understanding. OMT has traditionally been based on osteopathy concepts, which emphasize the body's ability to repair itself and maintain equilibrium. However, the use of cutting-edge technologies, such as sophisticated imaging and biomechanical analysis, has enabled practitioners to fine-tune their approaches in a more accurate and evidence-based manner. For example, the use of computer-aided modeling and simulation tools has allowed practitioners to gain a better understanding of musculoskeletal dynamics and tailor OMT therapies to particular patient needs.

Furthermore, increasing neurophysiological research has shed light on the complex interactions between the musculoskeletal and neurological systems.

This understanding has resulted in the creation of neuro-centric OMT approaches that target specific brain circuits to reduce pain and improve general well-being. As our understanding of the neurological basis of OMT grows, the future promises ever more customized and successful treatments tailored to each patient's specific physiological profile.

<u>OMT in the Evolving Healthcare Landscape.</u>

OMT plays an increasingly important role in the changing healthcare scene. In an era where patient-centered treatment and holistic approaches are gaining popularity, OMT fits well with the attitude of addressing the underlying causes of illness rather than simply treating symptoms. As the healthcare system shifts toward preventive and integrative medicine, OMT is positioned to play a critical role in addressing and preventing a variety of musculoskeletal disorders.

Collaboration between OMT practitioners and other healthcare professionals is increasing, promoting an interdisciplinary approach to patient care.

The incorporation of OMT into standard medical practices is becoming regarded as a helpful supplement to conventional treatments. This transition is reflected in the expanding number of healthcare institutions that are implementing OMT services into their offers, demonstrating the technology's acceptance and usefulness in today's healthcare market.

Furthermore, the growing emphasis on patient empowerment and collaborative decision-making is consistent with the ideals of OMT. Patients are taking a more proactive approach to health management, looking for non-invasive and holistic treatments for musculoskeletal conditions.

OMT, with its patient-centered philosophy and emphasis on restoring the body's natural balance, is well-positioned to fulfill healthcare consumers' shifting expectations.

<u>Training and Education for Future OMT Practitioners.</u>

As OMT gains popularity, the demand for well-trained, highly talented practitioners grows.

The training and education of future OMT practitioners are critical components that will determine the field's effectiveness and credibility.

Traditional osteopathic medical schools are broadening their curricula to include the most recent advances in OMT procedures, ensuring that students have a thorough awareness of both the historical roots and current breakthroughs in the profession.

Hands-on instruction remains an important component of OMT education, allowing students to gain the palpation skills and physical dexterity needed for efficient practice. Simulation technology and virtual learning environments are increasingly being used in OMT teaching, presenting students with realistic scenarios to help them improve their diagnostic and therapeutic skills.

Furthermore, multidisciplinary training programs that expose OMT students to collaboration with specialists from other healthcare disciplines help to promote a more comprehensive approach to patient care.

The growth of OMT education also entails remaining current on the newest research and evidence-based techniques. Encouraging research activities inside osteopathic institutions and encouraging cooperation with research-oriented medical institutes help to strengthen the evidence base for OMT.

This dedication to continued education and research ensures that future OMT practitioners are well-equipped to handle the complexity of modern healthcare and make important contributions to patient well-being.

CONCLUSION

Osteopathic Manipulation Therapy's future offers enormous promise as it advances in techniques, integrates into the shifting healthcare scene, and educates and trains future practitioners.

The continual refining and development of OMT procedures, which incorporate technological breakthroughs and a better understanding of neurophysiology, establishes this treatment approach as a dynamic and changing field within the larger healthcare context.

As OMT gets recognition and acceptance in mainstream healthcare, its place in preventative and integrative medicine is projected to grow.

The joint efforts of OMT practitioners and other healthcare providers represent a move toward a more holistic and patient-centered approach to musculoskeletal health.

The increasing empowerment of patients to manage their well-being is consistent with OMT's holistic concept, making it an excellent alternative for people seeking non-invasive and individualized interventions.

Training and educating future OMT practitioners is critical to the field's sustained growth and success. Osteopathic medical schools and training programs play an important role in preparing students with the information, skills, and ethical foundations required for effective and compassionate OMT practice.

The combination of sophisticated technologies, simulation tools, and interdisciplinary training strengthens the competencies of future OMT practitioners, preparing them to meet the changing demands of healthcare.

In essence, the future of osteopathic manipulation therapy is at the crossroads of tradition and innovation. OMT, which is based on osteopathy principles, is constantly adapting and evolving to incorporate new scientific knowledge and technological breakthroughs.

As it becomes an integrated component of the healthcare ecosystem, OMT has the potential to greatly improve individuals' well-being by addressing musculoskeletal disorders in a comprehensive, patient-centered, and evidence-based manner.